The Migraine Enigma

A Concise Explanation with Physician and Patient Perspectives

Stephen Landy, MD and Shoshana Y. Cenker

ISBN 979-8620893843

Printed in the U.S.A.

The Migraine Enigma

A Concise Explanation with
Physician and Patient Perspectives

FOREWORD 1

Dr. Stephen Landy has written a remarkably readable and extremely accurate book full of facts for headache patients about migraine — with a novel twist: There is a patient perspective in every chapter. No book has ever read like this one! There have been books written by doctors for doctors or for patients, and books written by migraine patients for patients — but this book written by a well-known and seasoned headache specialist, gives the reader both sides in each chapter.

Dr. Landy has dedicated his entire career to researching headaches and treating headache patients. You immediately sense how he speaks with his own patients when you read how he speaks to the reader. As a migraine patient, you'll like this guy. You will love how smoothly he conveys his information and wisdom, gleaned from years of speaking engagements, writing medical papers, research and close patient care.

Stephen's first chapter tells the reader all about himself — and at first, you might wonder where it's going and whether the book will help you to understand and improve your own headaches. You quickly realize the answer is a resounding 'Yes!' An academic neurologist trained in high-level institutions, he has done clinical research, plus academic writing and publishing and treated countless patients for over 30 years. You immediately recognize where his empathy for patients comes from when you read about him and how he feels about his patients.

Then you hear from his longtime patient, Shoshana, and read about her life with migraine, the prolonged, painful lack of diagnosis and proper treatment and her perspectives on all of it. You get her take in each chapter and it is riveting.

You learn all sorts of facts from Stephen Landy that you never knew, in a most palatable way, and you'll learn about the top headache clinicians and researchers in the world who have influenced him along the way.

Everyone wants to jump to the treatment chapter to find out how you can feel better, but don't miss the earlier chapters that explain what you need to know to understand your own headache issues. The treatment chapter is chock-full of critical information you need. Best of all, you come away from it understanding your disease intimately, where it fits in your life and what you need to do for yourself — with the help of your healthcare provider — to get the right outcome. You won't find a 10-step cure for your migraine. Instead, you'll come to grips with your disease and know if you are on the right track for a better result. Importantly, you'll realize if your doctor is the right one for you, or if you need someone different.

In the Migraine Resources and Support chapter, you'll learn where to get more help for yourself. After reading this book, I know you will have a better perspective of your disease and how well you have stayed on or strayed from the path to conquering your headache. If your headache trip has been like most, you have strayed from the ideal path a bit or been led to it by healthcare professionals. This book will educate you and help you to find the ideal direction going forward.

Alan M. Rapoport, MD

Clinical Professor of Neurology, The David Geffen School of Medicine at UCLA
Past President of The International Headache Society
Founder and Director-Emeritus of The New England Center for Headache

FOREWORD 2

Dr. Landy is a die-hard headache doctor who has made a difference in the lives of thousands and thousands of patients in one small region of the U.S., where headache specialists are a rare commodity and migraine patients can spend years before finding the one right doctor. He's given up the seemingly lucrative life of traveling from meeting to meeting and advisory board to advisory board for the privilege of diagnosing, treating and, eventually, helping scores of patients day-in and day-out. He has the opportunity to hear it all, see it all, try it all, fail it all, experience it all and, consequently, let patients teach him what no medical school, residency, fellowship or scientific meeting can possibly do.

Defining very carefully his goals — to reduce migraine patients' unnecessary suffering during their journey to help — Dr. Landy opted to share what he's learned in the past 30 years by adopting a writing style that non-medically educated migraine patients can readily comprehend. In essence, this book is a *migraine patient guideline.*

Brilliantly, Dr. Landy has teamed with Shoshana Y. Cenker, a migraine sufferer herself, who is also a very talented writer (a professional content writer, editor, proofreader and copywriter). Together, they author a first-of-a-kind book in which each chapter consists of two very distinct parts: one that is written by a well-educated and knowledgeable top-notch headache expert, whose understanding of migraine pathophysiology and its implications to a correct diagnosis and treatment is mature, conservative and up-to-date; and a second one written by someone who is by now well-educated and knowledgeable about the long and tortuous journey patients must take from first headache to proper diagnosis and treatment.

By acknowledging the many challenges of treating migraine, by recognizing that migraine is more than just a headache, by understanding that there is more than one pathophysiology to migraine, Dr. Landy encourages patients to remain positive and hopeful when different treatment approaches fail — and to trust that there is a treatment solution unique to them as individuals even if it may not help others.

Perhaps the most impressive and valuable part of the book is how Dr. Landy addresses the need to help patients in real-world situations — in which treating an individual patient often goes beyond the current state of medical knowledge or evidence-based medicine — all while refining the art of setting treatment expectations correctly. I warmly recommend that migraine sufferers take the time to read this book with care and leave its pages with hope.

Rami Burstein, PhD
John Headley-Whyte Professor of Anesthesia and Neuroscience
Harvard Medical School Vice Chairman Neuroscience Department of Anesthesia and Critical Care

Table of Contents

Migraine Disease
BY THE NUMBERS

PREVALENCE

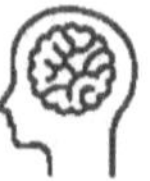

1 BILLION
people have migraine
disease/disorder worldwide

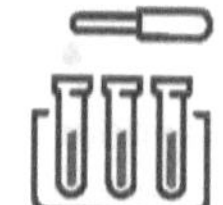

Migraine is most common
between the ages of

18 AND 44

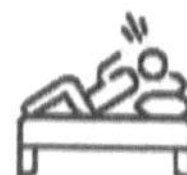

90%
of sufferers are unable to
work or function normally
during their migraine

NEARLY 1 IN 4
U.S. households includes
someone with migraine

Migraine is so common.
it affects as many as

50 MILLION PEOPLE
in the U.S. alone

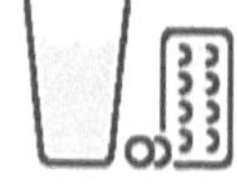

1 IN 6
Americans has migraine.
that's 12% of U.S. adults

Attacks usually last
between

4 AND 72 HOURS

Migraine is the

3RD MOST
COMMON DISEASE
in the world

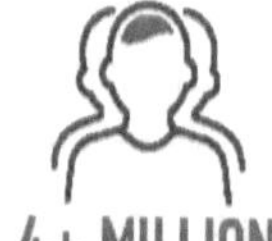

4+ MILLION
people have chronic daily
migraine = at least 15
migraine days per month

MIGRAINE-RELATED HEALTHCARE SPENDING

The yearly economic cost of migraine
in the U.S. alone is

$78 billion!

That translates to $9,000 annually for people with
chronic migraine and $2,000 for people with
episodic migraine, which includes healthcare
resource use and lost productivity and wages.

HOW OFTEN?

Every 10 SECONDS, someone in the U.S. goes to the
ER complaining of head pain, and ~1.2 MILLION visits
are for acute migraine attacks.

Migraine affects about 28 MILLION WOMEN in the U.S.
85% of chronic migraine sufferers are women
~10% OF SCHOOL-AGE CHILDREN suffer from migraine, and
up to 28% OF ADOLESCENTS between the ages of 15-19

PREFACE

You'll notice our book isn't the typical migraine book. And we think that's a good thing.

Not only do we have the neurologist/headache specialist's perspective, backed up by years of clinical experience and research, but within each chapter, we've also included the migraine patient's perspective (shown in a different font for helpful differentiation).

Each chapter represents clinically relevant migraine information, which serves as a practical and, hopefully, solid educational foundation for anyone who is either directly or indirectly affected by migraine.

Creating a solid foundation is frequently the key to future success, and we hope this book accomplishes this in an efficient, entertaining format. Each chapter focuses on different important migraine topics — and depending on your baseline migraine knowledge level and interest — they have different applicability from reader to reader.

The migraine pictures and captions at the beginning of each chapter illustrate the chapter's essence, and the artistic book cover was created to depict migraine in a creative and realistic fashion. We want to acknowledge and thank Barbara

Britt, a chronic migraine patient from Lexington, Tennessee, who has contributed the book's original chapter and cover art.

Many thanks as well to our proofreader extraordinaire Jamie Cameron for her keen eyes and expert editing skills, and our incredibly talented graphic designer and art director Faith Cohen for the infographic and promotional materials. And, so much gratitude to Charleen Davis, wise guide of all things books and publishing.

We also want to give special thanks to Drs. Burstein and Rapoport for thoroughly reviewing the book and each graciously writing their own forewords for *The Migraine Enigma*. They have both contributed mightily to the rapidly increasing awareness and understanding of migraine worldwide.

We're hopeful that all who read this book — patients, healthcare providers, students in the medical field, patients' family members, friends and employers — can relate to and better understand the important migraine information we're conveying. In other words: anyone directly or indirectly affected by migraine disease will benefit. We believe our unique format offers a valuable approach — one that's helpful to everyone.

At the end of this book, we've included a few pages for you to document your own migraine journey. As you're reading *The Migraine Enigma*, we encourage you to write helpful notes based on info from our book and your own thoughts and ideas that you can discuss with your provider in hopes that you reach a healthy migraine outcome and share it with family members and colleagues to convey your own migraine truth.

Chapter 1

The Migraine Healthcare Provider:

Stephen Landy, MD

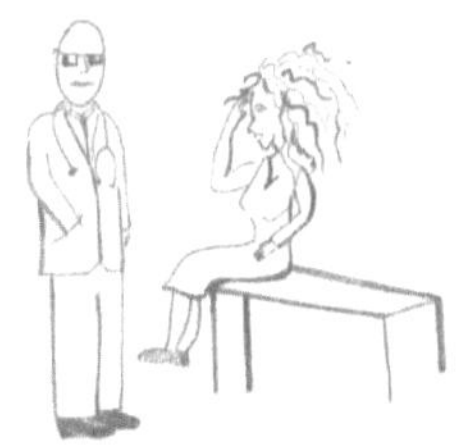

We know that the migraine healthcare provider evaluates and treats migraine patients. This person should ideally have an interest in migraine disease — preferably a special interest — and be capable of obtaining a thorough history of the migraine patient's migraine journey from its onset to the present clinical encounter.

The provider should also understand the unique characteristics of each migraine patient's presentation — such as previous treatments, the patient's understanding of migraine, migraine-related disability, comorbid conditions and their expectations, including treatment preferences.

Realizing that there is a spectrum of migraine headache from patient to patient — and even in the same patient from attack to attack — is paramount not only from a migraine diagnostic standpoint but also from a treatment standpoint. The provider should have adequate time to devote to uncovering these important details that are critical to implementing a quality treatment plan and developing an active migraine patient/provider relationship, resulting in shared decision-making (SDM). SDM is a key component of patient-centered healthcare. It is the epitome of clinicians and patients working together to optimize patient outcomes. In other words, both the patient and physician contribute to the medical decision-making process.

Here is my extensive journey of becoming a migraine provider.

I have devoted the 30+ years of my neurology career primarily to providing healthcare to migraine patients throughout Tennessee, Arkansas, Mississippi, Missouri, Alabama and Kentucky. I am board certified in neurology and headache medicine and a fellow of the American Academy of Neurology and The American Headache Society.

My professional migraine experience began in 1986 after I completed my neurology residency at Vanderbilt University in Nashville, Tennessee, and accepted a neurologist position at the Neurosurgical Group of Memphis in Memphis, Tennessee, where I attended and graduated from the University of Tennessee Medical School.

Along with evaluating general neurology patients, I was asked by a senior neurosurgeon partner to direct a headache clinic. Initially, I was overwhelmed by the tremendous number of undiagnosed migraine patients, some of whom were previously misdiagnosed — and the vast clinical spectrum of their respective migraine symptoms. I began to notice how disabled these patients were and how migraine was frequently associated with disability and a remarkable decline in quality of life.

The biggest surprise, however, was what I either overlooked or was not taught in medical school or during my neurology residency: even when the migraine diagnosis was made — the abortive and preventive migraine treatments were not optimally effective and were associated with unpleasant side effects.

So, in 1992, I became involved in migraine clinical research. Our headache center, Wesley Headache Clinic in Memphis, was a study site for a pharmaceutical company that initiated a multicenter emergency department research trial for the acute treatment of migraine. This new breakthrough of a migraine-specific medication, Imitrex, was approved by the Food and Drug Administration (FDA) later that year. It was a career-changing event for me and a life-changing event for many of my patients.

Imitrex became a first-line, migraine-specific symptomatic treatment for millions of migraine patients worldwide. Instead of symptomatically treating migraine headache with nonspecific medications, such as aspirin, ibuprofen and caffeine, alone or in combination, we could now treat migraine patients' pathology more specifically. This led to better treatment outcomes, increased awareness and diagnosis of migraine — and last but not least, more professional fulfillment.

It also cemented my professional career transformation to primarily practicing headache medicine with a main focus on migraine. After all, I attended medical school with the goal of helping people physically and mentally feel better and became a neurologist because I grew up with a fantastic big brother who unfortunately had cerebral palsy.

After six years of evaluating and treating this disabled group of migraine patients, I felt committed to addressing and improving this unmet migraine diagnostic and treatment need.

And there was improvement: Enhanced treatment outcomes included faster and more complete, consistent and sustained pain relief; mitigating migraine-related nausea and light and sound sensitivity; decreasing migraine-related disability, including less loss of work, social and personal time; and improved quality of life.

In 2003, I authored a medical manuscript entitled "Headache in the Workplace: An Evaluation of the Impact of Educational Programming on Employee Disability" published in the journal, *Headache & Pain*. This research was conducted at FedEx Corporation in Memphis and included 268 employees. The study demonstrated that worksite-based educational initiatives can improve the pain and disability of migraine, and migraine patients' quality of life. It also suggests that work productivity and absenteeism may be positively influenced by educational programs.

One research study led to the next and, over the years, our headache clinic's mission grew from just evaluating and treating migraine patients to participating in migraine research and education.

In recent years, I have directed the Baptist Memphis Neurology Subspecialty Headache Clinic and presently practice headache medicine in Tupelo, Mississippi — birthplace of Elvis Presley and my wife. Throughout my professional career, I have published more than 100 peer-reviewed journal articles and book chapters related to migraine. I have also functioned as Clinical Instructor, advancing to Clinical Professor of Neurology at the University of Tennessee Medical School.

I have been fortunate to witness the FDA's approval of migraine-specific abortive and preventive medications, which have enhanced migraine treatment outcomes. In 1988, the International Headache Society published headache classification criteria, which, with improved understanding of migraine pathology, have also enhanced our ability to complete high-quality migraine research and diagnose and treat migraine patients more effectively.

The pharmaceutical industry has contributed greatly to the discovery of migraine-specific medications, including triptans, calcitonin gene-related peptide (CGRP) antagonists and a ditan, for the abortive and preventive pharmacological treatment of migraine.

My migraine practice, including patient care, research, publication efforts and migraine education, has resulted in great professional satisfaction by affording me the fortuitous opportunity to evaluate and treat thousands of disabled, refractory migraine patients. I plan to continue in this field, both in research and treating patients, in an effort to provide insight, guidance and relief to migraine patients. I'm confident we will make many more migraine breakthroughs, which will result in improved patient satisfaction.

The remaining chapters of this book focus on migraine topics and information that are clinically relevant to migraine patients experiencing migraine pain and disability, as well as the general public, medical school students and healthcare providers.

The Migraine Patient: Shoshana Y. Cenker

Back in 1998, I had just graduated from White Station High School in Memphis, Tennessee, at the age of 18 and started college at my first pick: Indiana University (IU) in Bloomington, Indiana. Life was good. I met amazing new people, my classes were incredibly interesting, and I was thriving. Until I wasn't.

Headaches that I'd occasionally experienced before suddenly and unexpectedly became more frequent. And more painful. So much more painful. And they lasted longer, too. Like most teenagers, I was kind of a know-it-all (and by "kind of," I mean definitely), thinking that most likely the headaches were due to the added stress of college, change in schedule and long nights studying (ok perhaps a smidge of late-night partying too). In other words, I didn't think much of it, and simply self-medicated with over-the-counter (OTC) meds like Aleve. When I realized how much Aleve I was taking in a day — far too many — I switched to a different OTC like Excedrin. When that didn't help, I changed to a new med. You can see this unhealthy cycle taking shape.

Not only had I unknowingly started a tragic cycle of rebound headaches with all the meds, but they weren't even helping with the pain. And at this point, the headaches weren't headaches anymore. They were ice picks jabbing me in the inner corner of my eye. Jackhammers pounding on my neck. Shards of glass spiking through my temples.

I didn't know it at the time, but my headaches had become migraines. I'd never experienced a full-blown migraine before — all I knew was that the pain I was feeling was the most debilitating pain I'd ever felt.

Waking up with a migraine and going to bed with a migraine, I was barely able to function at IU. When I spoke with my parents about my health, we immediately scheduled several doctor's appointments in hopes of figuring out what was happening to me. Remember, I didn't know at the time that I was experiencing migraines.

In the blink of a (painful) eye, I quickly went from a healthy college student to a scared 18-year-old, unsure of the medical condition that I had. When there's pain in your head, face and neck — you think the worst. Did I have a brain tumor? If so, was it operable? Is something wrong with my eyes? Will I go blind? Because I had no idea what was happening to me, I spiraled down the rabbit hole of unknowns.

My rational side tried to think practically — I had made several doctors' appointments, and I'd get a diagnosis. For sure, right? Hopefully, right? During a regular break from college, I went home for these appointments, cautiously optimistic.

The first was a routine checkup with my general practitioner. While that workup showed I was healthy, which was great of course, it provided no insight into what was ailing me. So, I moved on to the next appointment: an ENT. Perhaps my pain was sinus-related. After a full workup, that doctor also couldn't come to any conclusions as to where my pain was coming from.

From there, I went to an eye doctor. The pain was so severe around and in my eyes — maybe that's where we'd find out some helpful information. Yet again, I got the good news that my vision was perfect, and my optometrist saw no issues with my eyes. But I was still no closer to a diagnosis. From there, I went to see my dentist. Was TMJ causing the pain in my head and neck? Well, no TMJ, and once again, no other issues found. The good news/bad news scenario played on. After exhausting the typical doctors you might see to help determine a diagnosis, I went for the big player based on a doctor's recommendation: an MRI and CT scan.

Let me try to articulate how scary this process was: Obviously it's terrifying because what if they did, in fact, find a tumor? But now try to imagine me — an otherwise healthy young'un who's 5'2" on a good day — inside this giant, intimidating machine, hoping I remembered to take off all my jewelry, including my numerous earrings, for fear they'd rip a huge hole in my ear from being torn out by the magnetism. It was certainly a frightening experience I'll never forget and wish for no one. Fortunately, the results came back perfectly normal. Unfortunately, it meant I was still undiagnosed.

The breakthrough happened, however, when I was casually chatting with my friend's mother. Jane had asked how college was shaping up for me, and after sharing how amazing IU was, I also told her about the "headaches" I'd been experiencing and my many doctor appointments. I explained that the pain had actually become so bad, I was considering taking a semester off from college until I could figure out what the heck was happening to me.

I'm sure you've heard the saying, "It's all about who you know." Well, that describes my conversation perfectly. Because of my description, including nausea with light and sound sensitivity, Jane immediately said that what I was experiencing sounded like migraines, and she referred me to her neurologist who specialized in migraines. He had helped her tremendously.

For the first time in weeks, I remember feeling a sense of relief. Finally, someone not only understood my pain, but she pointed me in the direction for help. Right then and there, I called to make an appointment with Dr. Stephen Landy.

To say that meeting with Dr. Landy changed my life is not an overstatement. Not only did I finally receive the correct migraine diagnosis, but he sympathized with me — recognizing and validating my physical pain and long journey seeking help. With my diagnosis, I finally felt like I could breathe again — all my pain and concern of the unknown was being answered. I physically felt stress begin to vanish from my body.

After that initial appointment, I dove into my own research about migraines. I wanted to be a partner with Dr. Landy in my treatment — and to do that effectively, I needed to become an expert.

One of the first things I learned is that migraines are hereditary and more prevalent in women. And wouldn't you know that my maternal grandmother, mom and sister all suffered from headaches — and we know now — migraines. Not to the extent I had them, thankfully, but this condition clearly ran in my family. (With an incredible daughter of my own now, I pray she doesn't ever experience one. Unfortunately, as you'll read about in later chapters, migraines do affect kids.)

I went through numerous preventative medications, which included varying doses, and pain relievers for when I got a migraine, before landing on the right combination with Dr. Landy's guidance. I distinctly remember fighting with my health insurance company to approve additional doses of one of the medications that zapped the migraine when I caught it in time.

While certain foods, alcohol and inconsistent sleep patterns are common triggers for migraine sufferers, I discovered they aren't mine by keeping food and sleep diaries. My trigger: weather — specifically, the change in barometric pressure. I can tell you if it's going to rain two days in advance. (I should have been a meteorologist.) Springtime sucks and summertime is even worse.

I also used to get an aura a few moments before a migraine struck — little sparkles of light danced as glimmering dots before my eyes — providing me precious minutes in which to quickly take a pain reliever. While I don't get auras anymore, they certainly used to be part of my saving grace.

The migraines I didn't catch in time or those I had no warning for were miserable... causing indescribable pain. And when the pain did stop — one to four hours later — I felt like I had been run over by a semi-truck. Weak, lethargic, no energy, my limbs and body felt heavy. My brain felt foggy and slow. It usually takes me a full day to recover from a full-blown migraine.

And I'm never without my pain relievers. I have the meds everywhere — my car, nightstand, bathroom, office desk, kitchen junk drawer, wallet. I never know when a migraine will strike or threaten to strike, but you better believe I'm prepared.

Armed with a significant amount of information from Dr. Landy, as well as some online resources and books, plus the helpful combination of meds — I finally felt like I was managing the migraines instead of playing defense.

Back at college, I was functioning and even thriving again. But I'd always make sure to have an appointment scheduled with Dr. Landy when I was visiting home on a break from IU.

The more I learned about migraine, the more I discovered that most people don't understand them. At all. They don't understand the intense, knockout pain. When someone has a broken arm, they have a cast. And seeing that, I believe, makes it more tangible for people to better understand the pain associated with a broken bone. Not so with a migraine — which is most certainly not *just a headache*, as many people believe.

I remember several of my college friends not fully understanding how different a migraine is from a headache. "Why are you hiding out in your pitch-black room again for just a headache?" they'd question. But for one friend, her understanding completely changed when she experienced one herself. One night, a couple of our friends came racing down the hallway to get me — one of my sorority sisters was experiencing terrible pain in her head, temple and eyes. She was nauseous and light and sound were nearly unbearable for her. Obviously, she was suffering from a migraine. Of course, I sprang into action to help her through it. When she had recovered the next day, she came to thank me. I'll never forget the validation, appreciation and empathy she gave me: "I'm sorry," she said. "I didn't understand what you went through. I thought it was just a headache. I can't believe you suffer through those on a regular basis and still function. Thank you."

After I graduated college, I lived and worked in other cities, including Chicago, Washington, DC and Atlanta. In each new city, I'd find a new neurologist/migraine specialist to monitor my treatment.

When I became pregnant with twins, everything changed again because not all the meds I was on were safe for the precious cargo I was carrying. I had read that for 50% of pregnant migraine patients, the migraines actually improve during pregnancy. Of course, my first reaction was: Woohoo! Unfortunately, I fell into the other 50%, and my migraines got worse. The human body is rather remarkable and works in mysterious ways sometimes. But, obviously the safety and health of the babies I was cookin' was paramount. And as we superheroes do, I suffered through it. And of course, now having three healthy children — twin boys and a daughter — it's all more than worth it.

Today, I'm doing remarkably well. I'm fit and healthy. Now living back in my hometown of Memphis, I once again get to partner in my health with Dr. Landy. I feel like I have a handle on the migraines and know which meds work and how to better prevent and combat an attack.

In the spring and summer months, when barometric pressure is at its worst, Dr. Landy expertly administers nerve blocks once a month — two injections in my forehead and two in the back of my head — and they are incredibly effective at preventing my migraines and even lessening the pain and frequency when I do have an attack. No one likes needles — but I'll take these nerve block injections any day over a migraine. And thankfully, one of the newest preventative injections is also giving me relief — considering the plethora of preventatives I've tried over the years, this was a welcomed surprise.

It's not like I haven't tried other measures. Aside from the dozens of preventative medications, I've also tried acupuncture, Botox, craniosacral therapy, massage therapy, reflexology, physical therapy, a no-carbohydrate diet, and on and on — basically anything and everything that anyone suggested might help, I'd try. You never know what might work for you — each body is different.

With more awareness about migraines than ever, I'm hopeful that with continued research, we can finally get to the bottom of this horribly painful ailment for better preventative and other treatment measures. In the meantime, I'll stick with Dr. Landy and what works for me.

To all the migraine sufferers: I want you to know that we hear you — there's a whole global community of researchers and doctors and patients who know you're suffering. We get your pain. And just like there was help for me through trial and error, there is help for you. Here's to your good health, and mine.

"It's frustrating that I cannot explain to people what migraine feels like."

Note: The quotes at the end of each patient chapter are the expressions and thoughts from fellow migraine sufferers.

Chapter 2

Migraine: More Than Just a Headache

In 2002, my friends and colleagues, Drs. Stewart Tepper, Fred Sheftell and Alan Rapoport from the New England Center for Headache,

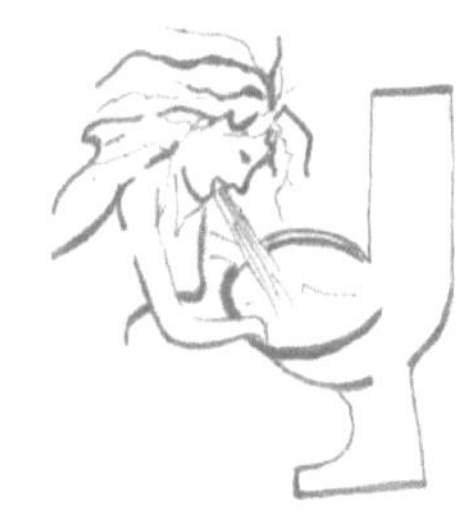

Throwing up. Yep, it happens. Often. It's gross, but to be expected.

published a migraine book called, *The Spectrum of Migraine.* They introduced this clinically relevant book by saying: While the common denominator is pain and disability, migraine presents in a variety of forms, with a variety of "faces."

The 19 chapters consist of the many different clinical presentations of migraine. I was fortunate to write the 17th chapter: "The Man with Headache and Weakness." In it, I describe one of my unfortunate patients with hemiplegic migraine. Hemiplegic migraine is a form of migraine characterized by weakness, which may mimic a stroke and almost always presents with transient paralysis of one side of the body, usually accompanied by migraine headache.

Migraine is more than just a headache. Frequently, people with migraine experience nausea, sometimes vomiting, as well as light, sound and smell sensitivity. Approximately 30% have a migraine aura that typically lasts five to 60 minutes and precedes the migraine headache. These aura symptoms are typically temporary visual disturbances such as flashes of light, blind spots, and/or other visual changes. Other less frequent aura symptoms include numbness, weakness and dizziness.

More frequent than aura, about 60% experience premonitory or prodromal symptoms a few hours or even a few days before the headache, which may include difficulty understanding and speaking, mood changes, fatigue, increased urination, diarrhea, increased thirst, repetitive yawning, insomnia, neck stiffness and food cravings. I vividly remember an initial evaluation of a migraine patient yawning incessantly when I walked into her examination room — I asked her if she was tired and she replied, "No, it's just the beginning of my migraine."

Migraine headache is relatively easy to diagnose, and I consider headache patients who have at least a one-year history of episodic, disabling headaches without other neurological complaints — except symptoms suggesting migraine aura — as having migraine headache.

Richard Lipton, MD, Professor of Epidemiology and Neurology and Director of the Montefiore Headache Center in New York City, and a team of migraine researchers have developed and validated a simple three-question screening survey called ID Migraine™. They reported that answering "yes" to two of the three simple questions effectively identifies migraine. The three questions are:

1. Has a headache limited your activities for a day or more in the past three months?
2. Are you nauseated or sick to your stomach when you have a headache?
3. Does light bother you when you have a headache?

In 1988, the International Headache Society (IHS) published the first International Classification of Headache Disorders (ICHD) and the ICHD-3 was published in *Cephalalgia*, the peer-review journal of the IHS in 2018. The explicit diagnostic criteria for migraine have diagnostic and research implications and have enhanced migraine research by frequently requiring fulfillment of these criteria before participating in migraine clinical research.

If you have migraine, it's important to count your monthly headache days — in addition to what you consider as a migraine headache day — because a person with migraine experiencing 15 or more monthly headache days typically has chronic migraine, which indicates more disabling migraine and a need for more aggressive and comprehensive treatment.

In other words, if a person has six tension-type headache days in a month and nine migraine days during the month, they have chronic migraine.

Unfortunately, Shoshana's arduous search for a correct migraine diagnosis is not uncommon. It is frequently misdiagnosed, undertreated and inappropriately disrespected. I have often jokingly referred to migraine as the "Rodney Dangerfield of neurological disorders," because of its frequent lack of respect by many healthcare providers, medical students, employers, work colleagues, families and friends.

Thanks to William Young, MD, neurologist and headache specialist at the Jefferson Headache Center in Philadelphia, I realize the importance of destigmatizing the migraine stigma. Merriam-Webster dictionary defines destigmatize as, "to remove associations of shame or disgrace," and I have personally witnessed the ostracization and isolation that innumerable patients with migraine incessantly experience because of discriminatory judgment and marginalization. Migraine preconceptions and misperceptions result in engendering the feelings of timidity, guilt, shame and embarrassment that many with migraine experience. Sadly, perception frequently drives reality, and it is our responsibility to change the mindset of many from their opinion, entrenched in ignorance or compassion fatigue, to an evidence-based opinion centered on our present knowledge and future migraine advancements.

The Grammy and Academy Award-winning song, "Shallow," beautifully performed and sung by Lady Gaga and Bradley Cooper depicts how migraine sufferers must sometimes feel because of their migraine disease and migraine stigma. Increasing awareness and legitimizing migraine — not as a weakness but instead as a respectable disorder — not unlike asthma and diabetes, will potentially help destigmatize migraine and encourage people with migraine to openly and candidly discuss their migraines as more than just a headache.

Migraine: More Than Just a Headache
Patient's Perspective

As a migraine patient, I appreciate that books like *The Spectrum of Migraine* and clinical papers are circulating, because their evidence helps inform doctors that migraine is not a one-size-fits-all issue. As Dr. Landy noted, the book says: …migraine presents in a variety of forms, with a variety of "faces."

In my 21-year experience suffering from (and now better managing) migraines, I can certainly speak to this. While my migraines are always painful and disabling, they often feel different, present in different ways and are constantly changing.

What does that mean? It means that I used to get an aura that would precede my impending migraine headache. Unfortunately, I don't anymore. It means my migraines used to begin with a sharp ice pick feeling in the inside corner of my eye; now, I usually begin to feel them in my neck. It means I used to feel nauseous every time a migraine would attack me, now I rarely do, yet I am still sensitive to smell, sound and light. Strong perfumes, IMAX movies and strobe lights are not my friends, but I learned to steer clear of those types of things.

In Dr. Landy's chapter "The Man with Headache and Weakness," from the helpful book *The Spectrum of Migraine*, he explains hemiplegic migraine. And although I have not suffered from that type of migraine and its one-sided symptoms, I now experience significant weakness and fatigue before some migraines, which is a new symptom that's creeped up only within the past year or so. What else varies? Sometimes my migraine will last a short time and get me first thing in the morning, while others beat me down for several hours in the evening.

All of this is to say that each migraine, each patient, each attack, each symptom can be different. We need doctors who have a firm grasp on these nuances to truly understand this challenging aspect of the disorder.

Dr. Landy and colleagues like him understand these crucial details and that many symptoms — some of which are beyond odd — fall away and new ones begin, oftentimes without any rhyme or reason. They are the unsung heroes because they *believe* us… and that's huge. Just because I've personally never experienced increased urination, diarrhea or repetitive yawning with migraine, for example, doesn't mean that the next patient who walks through his medical office doors doesn't or won't.

Migraine truly is an independent and ever-changing beast of a disorder.

Obviously, anyone who's ever suffered a migraine knows all too well that migraine is sadly so much more than just a headache. Conveying this to others who thankfully haven't experienced one can be difficult. (See the chapter on "My Migraine Journey" for a specific real-life account related to this very topic.)

Saying a migraine is just a headache is like saying a broken finger is just a papercut.

As Dr. Landy noted, all too often migraine is misdiagnosed, undertreated and not taken seriously. When I was finally correctly diagnosed with migraine by Dr. Landy for the first time in 1998 — after seeing countless other doctors in an effort to figure out what was happening to me — it was life-changing. And thanks to the ID

Migraine screening survey, correct migraine diagnoses are being provided sooner than later these days, which means patients can begin treatment and find relief sooner.

When I tell people that migraine is in the top 10 of most disabling medical illnesses in the world and the 3rd most common disease in the world, they are shocked — but again, that's a good thing. Sometimes people need to hear cold, hard stats to begin to get an awareness of the severity of migraine. We've certainly come a long way.

"I carry more guilt than you can possibly imagine about how my migraines affect the people around me."

Chapter 3

Migraine Prevalence, Gender Differences, Triggers and Pathology

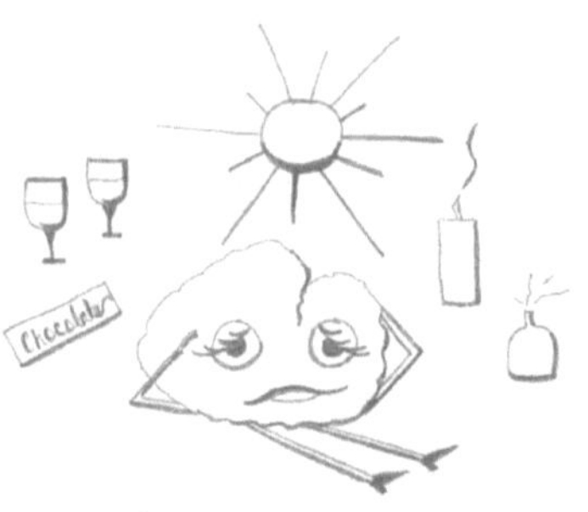

Anything can be a trigger. ANYTHING: food, alcohol, smells, sound, light, weather, sleep…

Migraine is a common disorder that is reported in migraine epidemiologic research in about 15% of the American adult population. It's at least two times more common in women than men and most common in middle-aged women during their most productive time of life. It's in the top five of most common diagnoses for an emergency room visit — over one million ER visits annually — and the number one reason for new patient neurology consultations.

Migraine is also common in children, occurring in up to 5% of boys and girls. In children, the migraine headache duration is sometimes shorter than in adults, 2–72 hours instead of 4–72 hours, and some children report migraine headaches lasting 10–20 minutes that are often less severe than adult migraines. Children occasionally present with abdominal pain, with nausea and vomiting, without headache. They also occasionally present with cyclic vomiting characterized by recurrent episodes of intense vomiting, at least four times per hour, separated by symptom-free intervals. Abdominal migraine and cyclic vomiting syndrome frequently are precursors to typical migraine headaches as the child matures, and these children and their parents have many times exhausted their resources before receiving appropriate diagnoses and effective treatment.

A number of factors may trigger migraines including hormonal changes in women, food and food additives, drinks, stress, bright lights, sun glare, loud sounds, strong smells, intense physical exertion, change of weather or barometric pressure and medications. Migraine triggers vary from person to person and, within the same person, from attack to attack. Most people with migraine have at least a few migraine triggers — and simply avoiding avoidable triggers may decrease their migraine frequency.

Many migraine patients tell me that exposure to more than one trigger concurrently is more likely to precipitate a migraine than one trigger alone. This is called by some, "trigger stacking," and I like to think of it as the perfect storm when explaining migraine triggers to patients. Unfortunately, some migraine triggers are unavoidable, such as weather change, but knowing their personal triggers may allow the person living with migraine to anticipate, prepare and possibly treat their migraines more effectively.

Migraine pathology is very complex, and the more I attempt to learn and understand its many complexities and phases, the more I realize what I don't know. Many brilliant scientists with different backgrounds have embraced and expanded our understanding of the pathophysiology of migraine.

In the 1980s, Michael Moskowitz, MD, at Harvard, eloquently described the neurogenic inflammation of migraine proving that the trigeminal nerve — a nerve that is responsible for head and facial sensation — transmits headache pain from blood vessels covering the brain. Migraine triggers activate this trigeminovascular system, causing pain and release of biochemical mediators that affect other areas of the brain that are responsible for the perception of migraine pain.

Based on my rudimentary explanation of Dr. Moskowitz's research, I sometimes simply explain to patients and colleagues that if you were to peel back the scalp, drill a hole through the cranium and look down over the covering of the brain during a migraine headache, it might look like hives. This simplistic and, hopefully, clinically relevant description of neurogenic inflammation enhances patients' and healthcare providers' understanding of migraine headache pathology.

Potentially, it allows them to understand the importance of treatment that may prevent the trigeminovascular-system activation and its significance relevant to mitigating migraine pain.

In the '90s, Rami Burstein, PhD, from Harvard and Academic Director of the Harvard Medical Faculty Physician Comprehensive Headache Center, began publishing his basic science and clinical practice experiences pertaining to migraine, central sensitization and cutaneous allodynia. I have had the fortuitous opportunity of collaborating with him through the years and have written two pertinent manuscripts about this migraine science: "Central Sensitization and Cutaneous Allodynia in Migraine" published in *CNS Drugs* and "Clarification of Developing and Established Clinical Allodynia and Pain-Free Outcomes" published in *Headache*.

Cutaneous allodynia is pain resulting from typically non-painful stimuli to normal skin such as discomfort combing your hair, shaving, wearing glasses, contact lenses, earrings or tight clothing. It's the surrogate clinical marker of central sensitization, which is a heightened excitability of the brain that may occur during a migraine headache. The migraine-induced neurogenic inflammation sensitizes brain cells in the trigeminal nerve pathway causing central sensitization that people with migrane may experience. The developing and established phases of central sensitization/cutaneous allodynia is a time-dependent physiologic event — and once migraine patients have established sensitization, they are less likely to respond to their symptomatic migraine treatments. This is scientifically why most physicians recommend that their migraine patients symptomatically treat their migraine headaches before they become moderate or severe.

The aura phase of migraine pathology is most likely secondary to a depression or slowing of brain activity followed by a reduction of blood flow, called cortical spreading depression — and this may serve as the catalyst for neurogenic inflammation and the subsequent migraine headache. The migraine prodrome most likely originates in the hypothalamus in many people with migraine who experience this. The hypothalamus is an area of the brain that coordinates activity controlling body temperature, thirst, hunger, sleep and emotional activity.

So, it's no wonder that many people with migraine experience these types of symptoms hours to days before their migraine headaches. The hypothalamic brain cells respond to changes in normal routine or homeostasis probably by activating the trigeminovascular system, thus potentially causing neurogenic inflammation.

This may explain "letdown" and weekend migraines triggered by a change in a migraine sufferer's normal routine, and was eloquently described in Roger Bannister's autobiography, *Twin Tracks*. He noted that after stressful elementary school weeks, "I had throbbing headaches nearly every Friday night, culminating in severe vomiting. No doctor was ever consulted, but, in retrospect, as a neurologist, I can diagnose that I had a variant of migraine." Interestingly, Sir Roger Bannister was the first person to run a mile in under four minutes.

Last but not least is the pathology of the migraine aftereffect, or postdrome, which I did not discuss in the previous chapter. The migraine postdrome in many clinical respects is similar to the migraine prodrome — except these symptoms occur after the migraine headache instead of before it. These symptoms include malaise, reduced concentration and melancholy. These symptoms that may pathologically represent the persistent brain changes of the migraine attack gradually resolve over a day or two. Yet again, it's no wonder many migraine patients tell healthcare providers and others that they are "worn out" after they have a migraine headache.

Considering the high prevalence and bewildering and potentially prolonged pathology of migraine, I am sure we will continue to unravel this complex and mysterious pathology.

Thanks to all the brilliant scientists who have, and are presently attempting to, unlock this intellectually challenging conundrum.

Migraine Prevalence, Gender Differences, Triggers and Pathology
Patient's Perspective

All the stats Dr. Landy provided in his chapter tell me something I had an idea about but wasn't certain of until seeing the evidence and data: People suffer from migraines. *Lots* of people — and especially women.

Why did I have a hunch about this? Way back in 1998, when I was first diagnosed with chronic migraine, I dove into research to learn as much as I could about this debilitating disorder. Not only did I seek out migraine societies for information, but I also reviewed case studies and newsletters. I consumed as much fact-based content as I could. Knowledge is power, of course.

And while those resources are incredibly important and helpful, it was actually in speaking to friends and family that I learned migraine's widespread impact on others. I had discovered that my maternal grandmother, mother and sister all suffered from migraine, though not as severe as mine. Clearly, it's more prominent in women and hereditary (thanks, fam!).

But as I began telling friends that I'd finally been correctly diagnosed, most often I'd hear something like: "Yeah, my mom has them, they're the worst!" and "I know a few people who have migraine pretty regularly." And just like that, the math of people affected was adding up in a spider web of migraine sufferers. It was like that silly game — "6 Degrees of Kevin Bacon" — everyone knows someone who suffers from migraine.

As Dr. Landy mentioned, studies show that just 5% of children have migraine. As far as I'm concerned, that's too many. Because I know that stat, coupled with the heredity and female prominence — even though my daughter is still young — I am hyperaware that migraine might get her one day. I watch for symptoms and truly listen when she says she has a headache. We must take children seriously.

Ahhh, triggers. It might sound odd — but thank goodness for triggers! It's a good thing that we are aware of the many triggers that exist. Some common, others not so much. I'm thankful because it's a big ole puzzle piece in the migraine prevention puzzle. By knowing your triggers, you can avoid them (well, some of them). Simple as that.

Strong smells are your trigger? Toss the perfume or cologne and even consider not cooking foods that produce strong smells, like fish. You love to cook fish? I hear you, but you know what you probably hate more? A terrible migraine. (Maybe just order that dish at your favorite restaurant.) Light sensitivity? Skip the IMAX movie. Alcohol gets you every time? Put the wine glass down, it's just not worth the pain.

Sure, it's annoying and a Debbie Downer to have to be so careful about triggers and not partake in some activities, foods or drinks, but I bet you know as well as I do that the alternative is much worse.

When I was first diagnosed, Dr. Landy advised me to keep a migraine diary that included when the attacks came on, how long they lasted and the severity. But he asked me to add in other details about my day — including how much sleep I got, and when I went to bed and woke each day — but most notably: what food I ate and when.

See, some of the most common triggers are certain foods: cheese, chocolate, nuts, wine (just to name a few). I kept my migraine diary and discovered that foods are not my trigger, but it was also good to rule out those potential triggers. And because our bodies are always changing, I go back to writing a food diary occasionally to check in and make sure a new food trigger hasn't popped up (especially after having children because of the unbelievable changes a woman's body goes through before, during and after pregnancy).

Gosh, how I used to love a rainy day. But I've learned that the weather and its changes in barometric pressure (though I have no issues on airplanes) are my migraine kryptonite. I should have been a meteorologist — I know if it's going to rain two days in advance. When I begin to feel tension in my neck, weakness, fatigue and the typical migraine "starter" pain in my head and eyes, (I check the forecast, who doesn't like to be proven right?!), and then proactively take my migraine-relieving prescription medicine.

Catching a migraine attack early is huge. When I do, I've found that the pain usually doesn't get worse and actually begins to subside. If it does progress, it's typically less intense and doesn't last as long, had I not caught the migraine early.

Early intervention is key. And that's why I carry my meds everywhere with me. *Everywhere...* my car, my wallet, nightstand, I even leave a small stash at the houses of my friends and family. Be prepared and be self-aware to recognize the beginnings of what could be a potential attack. An interesting new clue I've noticed starts in my neck — it feels like I need to pop or crack my neck. If I can crack it, I'm good. If I can't, a migraine attack is likely to come. Interesting, right? And weird — but incredibly helpful.

As we mentioned before, migraines can routinely feel different and present differently, but there are valuable clues for us to pick up on that help us see the patterns so we're able to manage migraine better. An interesting new clue I've noticed starts in my neck — it feels like I need to pop or crack my neck. If I can crack it, I'm good. If I can't, a migraine attack is likely to come. Interesting, right? And weird — but incredibly helpful.

After a full-on attack, I definitely experience the migraine postdrome Dr. Landy talked about. I describe it as feeling like I've been run over by a Mack truck. I'm exhausted, lethargic and feel like I'm moving in slow motion — physically and mentally. It takes a whole day, sometimes two, for me to recover. But knowing this helps me plan my day accordingly.

So, I'll leave all the medical science behind how triggers trigger (yep, I said it) migraine to the genius doctors. But, I'm grateful that this info, as well as the various phases of migraine and its pathology, is better known and well-circulated now. And even though I only understand a small fraction of the details about neurogenic inflammation, brain cells and blood vessels in the trigeminal nerve pathway, central sensitization and the trigeminovascular system — I believe it's important that patients have some understanding of the science. (But how to spell all of that?! Well, good thing there are online medical dictionaries.)

I'll say it again — knowledge is power — so arm yourself with as much as you can.

"A migraine is not a headache. It's a neurological exploding party in your brain that, unfortunately, pain happens to be invited to."

Chapter 4

The Spectrum and Comorbidity of Migraine

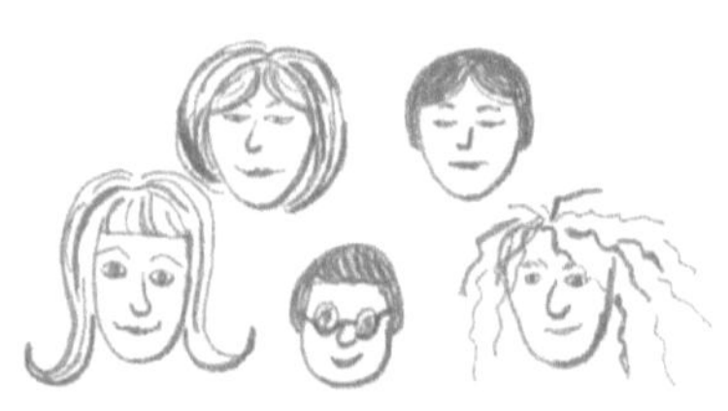

Through the years, it's been fascinating and **We all have migraine. But just as we are different, migraine can be different for each of us too.** clinically stimulating to observe the many different patient presentations of migraine and its various comorbidities. Not only do migraine symptoms differ from patient to patient and in the same patient from attack to attack, migraine patients differ in their various comorbidities. Comorbidity is when two illnesses occur at a greater than coincidental rate than what is expected, suggesting a relationship between the two illnesses.

Migraine comorbidities include depression, anxiety and bipolar disorders, restless leg syndrome, obesity, fibromyalgia, asthma and irritable bowel disease. Awareness of these comorbidities is an important consideration in providing optimal care from diagnostic and treatment perspectives. Typically, it's not good medical practice to recommend treatments that may exacerbate comorbid medical problems. Multimorbidity, defined as the co-occurrence of two or more chronic conditions, should also be addressed and treated judiciously.

The spectrum of migraine usually denotes the various symptomatic presentations of migraine rather than migraine frequency, but the migraine frequency spectrum is also patient-dependent and can change from week to week, month to month and year to year. Understanding the symptomatic frequency spectrums of migraine has diagnostic and treatment implications.

From a diagnostic perspective, it's important not to overlook migraine when patients present with episodic disabling headache brought on by weather change associated with runny nose and nasal congestion or when people with migraine present with headache triggered by stress that is associated with neck pain or tightness. These are frequent presentations of migraine headache, and approximately 80% of migraine patients with these sinus-like or tension-like symptoms have previously been diagnosed with sinus or tension headache, respectively.

Most people with migraine have less than four days a month of migraine headache, but unfortunately, about 40% have more than four days per month of migraine headache and have significantly more migraine-related disability. These people who experience the pain and disability of migraine require considerably more aggressive evaluation and treatment.

Last but not least is the person with chronic migraine who has headache at least 15 days a month, which on at least eight days have the features of migraine headaches. The chronic migraine population represents 10% of all migraine sufferers and is the most disabled and comorbid migraine group. This is the unfortunate migraine subset that makes up more than 50% of my patient population, and the ones who are frequently evaluated and treated at headache clinics throughout the United States.

Consideration of age and gender are also clinically relevant regarding the spectrum of migraine. I published a paper in *Neurology*, the peer-review journal of the American Academy of Neurology entitled "Migraine Throughout the Lifecycle. Treatment Through the Ages" stating that, "Clinicians who treat migraine must be aware of considerations specific to children, women and the elderly." Migraine variants should be considered in difficult-to-diagnose children who are diagnosed with benign paroxysmal vertigo, paroxysmal torticollis and cyclic vomiting. Adult and adolescent females frequently have menstrual, pregnancy, menopause and estrogen supplementation relationships to their migraines — and even though migraine typically declines in the elderly, it's still quite common: 8% of women and 3% of men over 60 years of age. The elderly patient may also present with late-life migraine accompaniments that resemble symptoms of stroke but are migraine-induced.

Considering the multifaceted components of the migraine spectrum and comorbidities allows the patient and clinician to improve diagnosis and, ultimately, to individualize and recommend a tailored approach to the patient's treatment plan. The goal is always to reduce migraine frequency, optimize symptomatic and preventive migraine treatment, reverse migraine-related disability and improve the patient's quality of life.

The Spectrum and Comorbidity of Migraine
Patient's Perspective

In his section of this chapter, Dr. Landy noted that migraine symptoms differ from patient to patient and in the same patient from attack to attack, and there are various comorbidities. I have lived with and can speak to all of this. To break it down to simple terms, migraine is basically a crapshoot. It's not a black-and-white condition, there is so much gray area that it continues to remind patients, doctors and researchers to expect the unexpected.

Since I've already touched on many of these aspects in previous chapters, here's a quick recap of some of it.

Patient-to-patient symptom differentiation: As I mentioned, several of my family members suffer from occasional migraine, as do some friends. When we sit around talking about new treatments or the latest research (I know, we're super cool), we inevitably share details of some of our recent attacks.

While we have some symptoms in common like light, sound and smell sensitivities, there are others that we don't share — most notably where the pain occurs and how it feels can be different. Now, my pain usually begins in my neck; my friend's attacks the inner corner of her eye; a relative feels it at the base of the back of her head. I describe my neck pain as tightening, gripping, heavy pressure; my friend describes hers as a shard of stabbing glass; my family member says it feels like a jackhammer banging on her skull. What's interesting, just as Dr. Landy described, is that I know what they're feeling. My attacks and symptoms have changed over the 20+ years I've suffered from migraine, but I've experienced the exact same pain at some point during that time.

Allow me to use a well-known movie quote that might better articulate these two important points about migraine — the patient-to-patient and attack-to-attack differences: "Life is like a box of chocolates, you never know what you're gonna get." Thank you, Forrest; it's true for so many things. (And if chocolate is your trigger, maybe stay away from the box.)

As far as the comorbidity aspect goes, this too applies to me and friends and family, though I'll just speak to mine.

In addition to migraine, I have suffered from depression and insomnia. Depression is comorbid with migraine, and Dr. Landy has told me that insomnia is associated with more frequent and severe migraine.

I've learned that it's so important for your migraine doctor to know any and all ailments you have in addition to migraine. There's no shame here — it's only in your best interest. Why? As it turns out, there are several medications that can be used to treat one condition but also may help with another ailment.

For example, there are antidepressants and muscle relaxers that may also help with migraine prevention. I like to call that a twofer. The trifecta might be an antidepressant effectively treating depression, insomnia and migraine or a muscle relaxer relieving muscular discomfort, insomnia and migraine. Here's what's important: When your doctor knows all the illnesses you suffer from, he/she is better equipped to provide you better treatment. Is it embarrassing to talk with your doctor about irritable bowel syndrome? Maybe. But they've definitely heard it before, and sharing those details can only help you. I mean, what's worse: sheepishly talking about your bathroom habits privately in your doc's office or suffering a full-blown migraine?

Dr. Landy also wrote about the migraine frequency spectrum, and this too fits right into that gray area. Sometimes, there is no rhyme or reason to why I'll have a wonderful full week without a migraine, but then the very next week they come back to punish me every other day. As we noted previously, triggers do play a role, but it often seems like migraine has a nasty mind of its own and doesn't play by the "rules."

My migraine has evolved over the years, and I expect it to continue to do so. Who knows exactly if and how I'll be affected by them when I reach menopause and older age — but knowing to expect some kind of change is better than nothing. Thankfully, there's more awareness and research about the devastating effects and changeable nature of migraine.

My takeaways from this chapter?

1.   You and your migraines are unique. What goes for you may not apply to another migraine sufferer. Know that even your own attacks can vary.

2.   Communicate with your healthcare provider. Make sure they know about even the slightest change in symptoms, frequency, triggers, other illnesses and medications. Here's where that new SDM recommendation, advocated by national headache organizations, comes into play: Be a partner with your provider, so together, you can be the most effective dynamic duo against your migraines.

"It's not just pain. It's a complete physical, mental and emotional assault on your body."

Chapter 5

Migraine Treatment

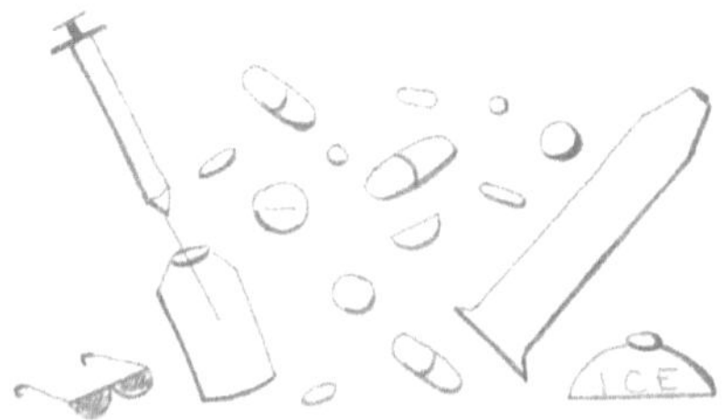

The treatment of migraine includes nonpharmacologic,

Sufferers will try ANYTHING to stop the pain. Pills, more pills, shots, ice, darkness...

acute and preventative pharmacologic options. Treating healthcare providers should address medication overuse versus medication-overuse headache (MOH). MOH potentially — and unintentionally — creates stigma by implying the patient is to blame for taking too much medication, so many experts prefer calling this medication adaptation headache or medication response headache. Consideration of the migraine patient's history in detail, including monthly migraine days and headache days, migraine-related disability, comorbidity, associated symptoms such as nausea, light, sound and smell sensitivity, previous migraine treatments, patient treatment preference and insurance coverage, are important to achieving optimal treatment outcomes.

Nonpharmacologic treatment of migraine includes avoidance of individualized trigger factors, behavioral modification, cardio exercise, nutritional supplements and acupuncture. Behavior interventions include relaxation techniques, biofeedback and cognitive-behavioral therapy. The expression "mind over matter," comes to mind, and these types of mind-body therapies have the potential to mitigate pain by changing the pain perception and physiology. Nutritional supplements such as magnesium, riboflavin and coenzyme Q10 have been effective in small clinical trials. Feverfew, melatonin and butterbur without alkaloids may also be helpful.

Neuromodulation with neuromodulatory devices is a relatively new nonpharmacologic approach in treating migraine. These devices turn down brain activity rather than activate it, and thus may turn down the hyperexcitability of the migraine brain. Presently, there are non-invasive devices approved by the FDA for migraine treatment, all with minimal risk. These include a transcutaneous supraorbital neurostimulator, neuromodulation patch, transcranial magnetic stimulator and non-invasive vagus nerve stimulator. There are other neuromodulatory devices on the horizon showing promise for migraine patients, including the Allay Lamp that incorporates a special narrow band of green light that is less likely to exacerbate migraine than yellow, blue and red colors.

Regarding acute pharmacologic migraine treatment, people with migraine want rapid, complete, sustained, consistent relief of migraine headache without side effects. Achieving these outcomes is sometimes unrealistic, but if patients consider different acute treatment approaches geared to their different migraines, they may be more likely to achieve these goals.

Almost 100% of people with migraine take medication — either over-the-counter or prescription medication acutely for their migraine headaches. People who take acute medication for their migraines on more days than not risk developing MOH. Differentiating medication overuse (MO) from MOH is challenging because as headaches accelerate in frequency, medication use also increases — and distinguishing whether MO is the cause or consequence of the patient's frequent headaches is important from diagnostic and treatment perspectives. Preventing MOH is a critical component of acute pharmacologic migraine management.

Education regarding proper use of acute or symptomatic medication assists patients in preventing MOH. This education includes instructing patients on optimal use of the acute treatments, including taking the right drug at the right time, at the right dose and the right formulation. In my experience, if offered and counseled on appropriate acute treatment options, patients quickly learn from their own experiences which acute medications are best for them. These options include nonspecific and migraine-specific medications.

Migraine-specific means the medication was developed specifically for migraines and, until recently, primarily referred to triptan medications. Triptans were first introduced in the 1990s in the United States and are readily available in tablet, nasal spray and injectable formulations. Other migraine-specific medications are now available, including CGRP antagonists and a ditan. Stay tuned, as more are on the way. Since migraine headache is frequently associated with nausea — and sometimes vomiting and allodynia may be present — non-oral formulations may be more helpful because they bypass the gastrointestinal tract, which results in more complete and faster absorption. Nonspecific migraine medications include many of the over-the-counter pain medications that frequently contain caffeine, acetaminophen and aspirin. Prescription analgesics include controlled pain medications and combination drugs, frequently with butalbital and caffeine.

A rational polytherapy is sometimes beneficial, such as combining a triptan with an anti-inflammatory medication, including ibuprofen or naproxen sodium.

Proper use of acute pharmacologic treatments is vital in optimizing acute migraine treatment outcomes. I frequently recommend attack-specific treatment, which obviously is different from patient to patient and within the same patient from attack to attack. The addition of an antiemetic may be beneficial.

Frequency of migraine and headache days, use of acute medication and migraine-related disability determine the need for migraine preventive pharmacologic treatment. Most likely, at least 50% of migraine patients are good candidates for migraine preventive treatment, and more than 80% of the patients I evaluate and treat for migraine are on migraine prophylaxis. Patients who have migraine at least four days a month, require acute medication on those days, and have impaired function at home, work or socially should discuss their need for migraine preventive therapy with their healthcare provider.

Until recently, migraine preventive medication options were primarily drugs repurposed for migraine — meaning they were medications initially intended for another medical indication and serendipitously found to be helpful for migraine. These repurposed medication classes include anticonvulsants, antihypertensives and antidepressants — alone or in combination. They may be helpful, but typically, because of lack of efficacy or intolerable side effects, patients discontinue them.

They should be started at a low dose and gradually increased over months until they either effectively decrease migraine frequency, intensity or duration, or cause significant unacceptable side effects.

In 2010, the FDA approved Botox for chronic migraine patients 18 and over — and even though this was repurposed from its original use — it's been a welcome advance for this very disabled and comorbid group of migraine patients. Anti-CGRP monoclonal antibodies specifically developed for migraine prevention have recently received FDA approval for adults. They are a major breakthrough for millions of migraine patients, allowing many to finally achieve reduction of migraine frequency, intensity and duration, with improvement in their quality of life, resulting in less migraine-related disability. In general, they are well tolerated.

Pediatric migraine preventative medication recommendations are less appealing than those for adults. The Childhood and Adolescent Migraine Prevention (CHAMP) Study, published in *The New England Journal of Medicine* in 2017, demonstrated increased side effects without decrease of migraine frequency and disability, comparing the most commonly prescribed preventative medications to placebo. All treatments reduced migraine frequency by 50% or greater and, interestingly, all patients received instructions about effective acute medication treatments and healthy lifestyle habits, including adequate hydration, sleep, exercise and regular meals with healthy eating. The attention to acute medication and nonpharmacologic migraine education may have accounted for the high placebo response, supporting the importance of education for pediatric migraine treatment.

If all else fails, nerve blocks of occipital and supraorbital nerves and the sphenopalatine ganglion and elsewhere are sometimes effective. Occasionally, intravenous fluids and intravenous or intramuscular medication at the patient's doctor's office, urgent care facility or emergency room can serve as a last-resort treatment that is frequently safe and effective.

I sometimes respond to refractory, disabled, desperate migraine patients when asked about other treatments by saying, "As long as it's effective and safe, why not try it." Thankfully, because of the tremendous scientific and clinical migraine advances, resulting in better, more specific migraine treatments, this question is asked much less often.

Migraine Treatment
Patient's Perspective

I actually have a lot to say about migraine treatment and that's because, thankfully, there are so many treatment options available. But I'll try to be concise.

Let's start with medications. I went through some trial and error, especially in the beginning, when figuring out the best treatments for me. And as it often goes with migraine (expect the unexpected, of course), over the years, some treatments stopped working and we'd begin the search for a new option. Plus, new treatment options come on the market from time to time.

Years ago, one of my mentors told me: "You always have options, some are just better than others." It's one of the best pieces of advice I've ever heard, and I'm reminded of it often. Though she was referring to business, it certainly applies to any facet of your life — including migraine treatment.

So, options are great and there are many for migraine. (Hooray!) Just remember that what works for you may not work for your mom. And what works for you now may not work for you later. And what works for one of your migraines might not work for the next. (Boo!) But you do have options.

For the first several years after my diagnosis, at the onset of a migraine, I took a medication for nausea along with another one for the migraine headache. (Eventually, nausea wasn't an issue for me anymore.) When the oral migraine medication stopped working, I tried a nasal spray. When that wasn't as effective, I switched to a patch. And now I'm back to an oral medication. (Triptans are my friend!) There are also injections and quick-dissolving medications.

My point is... there is medication that will ease your migraine headache and other symptoms related to migraine.

A word of caution, though. An all-too-common medication prescription is narcotics. Without speaking from both sides of my mouth — while I do believe that there are certainly patients who need and can be safely treated with narcotics — I must warn you about them with my own narcotic story. I'm not proud of it, but it's important to include in our book.

Long before the opioid crisis, when I was briefly under the care of a different neurologist while I lived in another state, I quickly became addicted to narcotics, specifically Percocet and Fentanyl. This doctor wrote me narcotic prescriptions lightning fast, and I happily filled them and popped the meds that not only stopped my migraine pain (albeit temporarily) but also gave me a high. As you can probably guess, I then had to keep upping the amount I was taking.

Addiction was swift and the fallout was disastrous. When I say that quitting narcotics cold turkey and going through withdrawal that lasted for several months compares in misery to a migraine, I'm not exaggerating. I got through it, but it was one of the most difficult life experiences I've ever had. I wouldn't want anyone to suffer the same.

So, yes, there is a place for safely using narcotics for migraine, but do so under the strict guidance of your responsible doctor and, even then, do so with caution.

Let me touch on other treatment options... I've tried acupuncture, craniosacral therapy, massage, physical rehab, biofeedback, downed supplements including magnesium and riboflavin, used a neuromodulation device, Botox and more. Unfortunately, those didn't offer me much relief, though I know people who have been helped by some of those options.

And even though it seems like a long list of fails in my case, I was and still am up for trying anything and everything that might help reduce the devastation of migraine. You never know if the next thing will happen to work. My advice: try each of them, one at a time, and maybe one (or more) will help you.

In his section of this chapter, Dr. Landy also spoke about overuse of medication. In addition to opioid overuse and misuse, overusing even over-the-counter meds and non-opiate prescriptions can cause medication-overuse headache, which in the past was called rebound headache. In the beginning, before I was able to manage my migraines better, I would get into a vicious cycle of rebound headaches. As Dr. Landy noted, education is critical and, thankfully, I quickly learned from my experience, but only with the help of his expert teaching and guidance.

On to preventatives. Wouldn't it be amazing if everything I've written about so far in this chapter was a moot point because of perfectly effective migraine preventative medications? Well, we're not there yet, but there are certainly some very helpful preventatives on the market now.

Throughout my migraine journey (you can probably guess where I'm going with this by now), I've gone through a few different preventatives. I've been on one seemingly helpful oral preventative for several years. And I'm now using a new migraine-specific preventative injection, which I inject into my thigh every 28 days (an anti-CGRP monoclonal antibody). Thankfully, it seems to be working — this is huge! I did try two other recently released preventative injections, which unfortunately didn't seem to help me — but I have heard they are helping others. And it makes me so happy to hear others finding relief.

So, if you're unsatisfied with your preventative, under the direction of your doctor, keep trying different options. This is important: Stick with each one long enough to determine if and when to call it a day with that med before moving on to the next.

In addition to my oral preventative and the new preventative injection, my miracle over the past year has been nerve blocks. I definitely don't enjoy the two needles being stuck in my forehead above my eyebrows and two more in the back of my head, but the roughly three weeks of reduced migraine I enjoy because of them is well worth it.

To be clear, I am not migraine-free, but the nerve blocks have worked better for me than anything else I have tried. And now with the addition of the new preventative injection, I'm living more migraine- and pain-free days than ever before. Some of my migraines even present differently now, though I didn't realize it at first. Rather than sharp, intense, unbearable pain, I sometimes feel exhausted, weak, listless. Eventually, it dawned on me — that's the result of the new preventative injection kicking in. I'll take sluggish over a giant cactus needle poking in my head any day!

One more note — about a seemingly small item with a big impact: WellPatch. When I'm down and out with a migraine, I lay one of these patches on my forehead and neck. It takes a few minutes, but when it begins to work, it burns so good. What do I mean? This little patch somehow gets so cold that it begins to numb the sharp and pounding pain. I have a stockpile of these bad boys in my bathroom closet. I encourage you to do the same.

Well, so much for being concise; it's time to wrap up this chapter. Just remember: You have options. Great options!

"Once the pain fades, it feels like I ran a marathon. My body — and my brain — are exhausted."

Chapter 6

Migraine Resources and Support

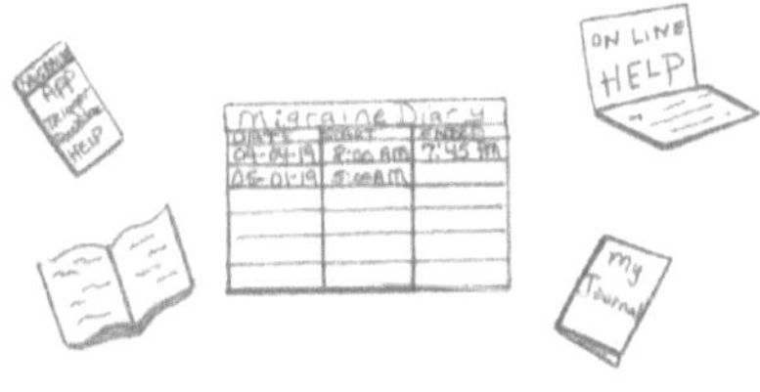

There are outstanding national and international **Write everything. Never stop looking for help. It's out there.** headache societies, which are excellent sources of migraine-related information and support the migraine population in many ways. For over 25 years, I have been a member of the American Headache Society, the International Headache Society and the National Headache Foundation. All three of these organizations actively educate healthcare providers and patients about migraine and offer support to anyone interested in improving the quality of life for all people with migraine.

The mission of the American Headache Society, which was founded in 1958, is to improve the care and lives of people living with headache disorders. Educating physicians, health professionals and the public, and encouraging scientific research are the primary functions of the society and its 1,500+ members.

Working alongside the American Headache Society is the American Migraine Foundation whose mission is to mobilize a community for patient support and advocacy, as well as drive and support impactful research that translates into treatment and advances for patients with migraine. Founded in 2010, it also provides global access to information and resources for people with migraine and their families and friends.

The International Headache Society (IHS) statement of purpose is to advance headache science, education and management, and promote headache awareness worldwide. With its 1,300+ members, the IHS is an international professional organization working with health professionals, the public, politicians, academic centers, insurance companies and other key stakeholders involved in migraine for the benefit of people affected by headache disorders.

The mission of the National Headache Foundation is to cure headache and end its pain and suffering. Its vision is a world without headache. To achieve its goals, it has increased public awareness regarding headache disease and its impact on the individual, their families and society. Since 1970, the organization has worked to advocate that headache and migraine are legitimate neurobiological diseases. The National Headache Foundation serves as a premier resource by providing information to patients, health care professionals and the media, and it supports research into the potential causes of headache disease and the development of new treatments.

I encourage all migraine patients and their families, employers, friends and colleagues to become actively involved in diagnosing and optimally treating migraine. Knowledge is power, and becoming more informed about the underpinnings of migraine, including its various treatments and disability, ultimately can make the migraine journey much more realistic and pleasant. These societies have been extremely beneficial to millions of migraine patients worldwide.

American Headache Society	americanheadachesociety.org
The International Headache Society	ihs-headache.org
American Migraine Foundation	americanmigrainefoundation.org
National Headache Foundation	headaches.org

**Migraine Resources and Support
Patient's Perspective**

Thankfully, we are living in an age in which information and help are just a click or phone call away. When I was first diagnosed, the internet was barely a thing, awareness of migraine was severely lacking and resources were difficult to come by. (I mean it was hard enough just to get someone to believe how devasting the pain was — pain that I endured on a regular basis.)

Not anymore.

There is a wealth of info, data, drug stats, treatment details, research, case studies and other resources online. And, all of the remarkable organizations Dr. Landy mentioned are championing the effort to help migraine sufferers in numerous ways. (Migraine sufferers, rejoice!)

But it gets better. These organizations aren't working in a vacuum. They're communicating and sharing information, studies and solutions — they're working together to help us. That's pretty amazing!

For me, it provides some relief to know that there are incredibly smart and talented people across the globe going to bat for me — trying to help me and fellow migraine patients. This tells me that these agencies understand my pain and are doing something about it. These organizations believe us when we say how debilitating migraine is. And they should be applauded for it.

Of course, in addition to those respected organizations, there are other agencies and countless support groups, plus informative websites, forums, discussion groups and other migraine-related resources that blanket the internet. Dive into them. Read, learn and share. Maybe something you learn today can help another migraine sufferer. Wouldn't that be great?!

What if you see or hear something questionable or worrisome or downright confusing? Simply bring it up with your doctor. Remember, communication is super important.

Just know this: You're not alone. Help is all around you.

"If you don't get migraines, you don't get migraines."

Chapter 7

Your Migraine Journey

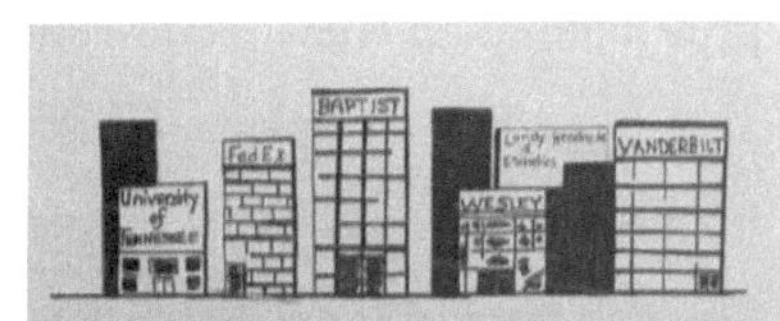

In Chapter 1, I mentioned the importance of capturing and elucidating the journey of people with migraine. This chapter is primarily a discussion of important components that will hopefully lead people with migraine to a more expeditious and comfortable journey. This is frequently accomplished by considering, uncovering and understanding the importance of each and every migraine patient's unique migraine story during all patient interactions.

Migraine is a polygenetic disorder — meaning there are multiple genes responsible for the many different phenotypic or clinical presentations of migraine. Migraine is also influenced by epigenetic susceptibility — meaning that your genes are capable of changing their function without changing their DNA sequence.

Epigenesis is the way a gene changes based on environmental influences, which can positively or negatively impact the way our genetic makeup is expressed. Epigenetic variance explains why identical twins with migraine, sharing identical genetic profiles, can have different migraine presentations and may require different treatment.

Genetic and epigenetic differences explain why it is impossible for any two people to be entirely alike — establishing the basis and importance of highlighting the unique migraine journey of each and every migraine patient.

Merriam-Webster's dictionary defines journey as an "act or instance of traveling from one place to another or something suggesting travel or passage from one place to another." One of my favorite bands, Journey, named by John Villanueva, who worked on the band's management team, obviously recognized the value of understanding and respecting the journey.

Most of us agree that good migraine healthcare requires the person to seek care, obtain a diagnosis and be prescribed appropriate treatment. I feel that this is the foundation of an appropriate migraine journey for most migraine patients. One publication entitled, *Barriers to the Diagnosis and Treatment of Migraine: Effects of Sex, Income, and Headache Features* and a second publication entitled, *Assessing Barriers to Chronic Migraine Consultation, Diagnosis, and Treatment: Results From the Chronic Migraine Epidemiology and Outcomes (CaMEO) Study* conclude that only 26% of episodic and 5% of chronic migraine people traverse these three barriers to care successfully. These dismal statistics may explain why many migraine patients unfortunately experience prolonged, burdensome, painful journeys.

My patients have amazed and amused me regarding their individual and unique migraine journeys. Their very personal information has helped me immeasurably to, hopefully, help them in their pursuit of correct diagnosis and optimal treatment with the goal of a more pleasant and less disabling migraine journey. Hearing a migraine patient say, "I am now in control of my migraines instead of them controlling me," fortunately has become a more frequent reality.

It has been a joy and a privilege writing this book with Shoshana. I appreciate and respect her willingness to transparently articulate and share her arduous migraine journey, which is hers and hers alone. I am sure many of you have experienced your own migraine journey, too. Expressing it may be cathartic and, hopefully, therapeutically beneficial. Quoting Jim Valvano, the former great NCAA basketball coach at North Carolina State: "Don't give up. Don't ever give up."

Your Migraine Journey
Patient's Perspective

In Dr. Landy's chapter, he uses medical terms that I can barely pronounce: polygenetic disorder; phenotypic; epigenetic. But, his explanation of those terms certainly makes sense, especially the interesting detail about identical twins — who have carbon copy genetic profiles — yet can have different migraine attacks and need different treatment.

Well, it just so happens that I have twin sons who are fraternal not identical, but I can still drive Dr. Landy's point home using them as pseudo examples. The way I describe my boys to people is this: "Yes, they're twins, but they are their own people — they're *individuals* who just happened to have shared a home together for nine months before they were born. They think differently, have incredibly different personalities, enjoy different foods and have different skills, strengths and weaknesses."

As we've stated throughout our book, every person's migraine experience is different — even identical twins.

While I feel like a broken record saying it again, this is clearly one of the themes of our book and of migraine: migraine is unique — there's no black and white; there's no box that migraine neatly fits into; there's no one-size-fits-all. And, as each migraine patient's journey is unique, their journey will likely change along the way. Mine sure has.

Unfortunately, compassion fatigue from medical providers is common — but it's something those of us with migraine can't and shouldn't tolerate. I'm grateful that doctors like Dr. Landy understand that info I share with him about my migraine experience at one office visit might be different at the next visit. Patients need to feel that they are believed, heard and taken seriously when their migraines change, including symptoms, triggers and response to treatment.

I'll even go a step further. Dr. Landy is also open to new ideas and suggestions I bring in during office visits. Remember how we've both mentioned how important education is? Well, I'm always reading about migraine health, and whenever I come across an article or blurb or ad about a new treatment or medication, we discuss it together. (Hello, SDM!) I feel like I'm a participant, not just a passive observer. After all, it's *my* migraine journey, right?

Dr. Landy has always listened to me over the many years, and it's refreshing to find an expert of his caliber who's receptive. I truly feel that he and I are partners in my migraine journey. That's the kind of patient-doctor relationship you want — one that benefits both of you. His expertise guides me for healthier, less painful days while the stories and info I share help him help me and, perhaps, other migraine sufferers too. It's a healing dance of give and take.

Together, our hope is for all migraine sufferers — in all of their uniqueness — to be able to live the healthiest, most pain-free lives they can.

"My migraine battle will continue, but I will not give up."

Chapter 8

Migraine in the Future

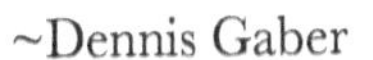

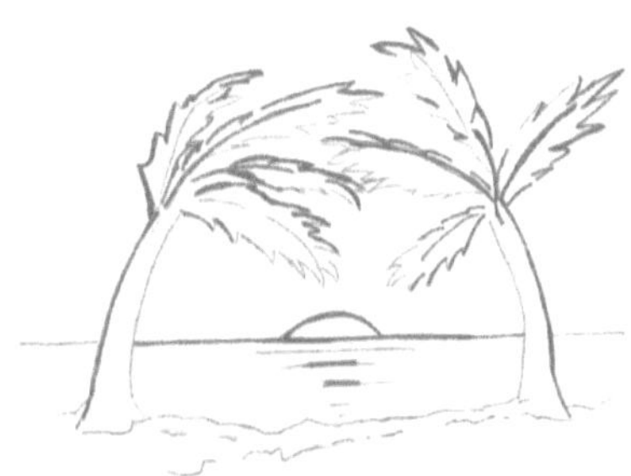

"The future cannot be predicted, but futures can be invented."

~Dennis Gaber

Nobel Prize in Physics, 1963

Since I am a believer that the past frequently predicts the future in direct and indirect ways and often is the catalyst for future breakthroughs, I predict the future of migraine is very bright.

The 1980s were pivotal years regarding our understanding of migraine pathophysiology, providing us the opportunity to understand the importance of neurogenic inflammation and a glimpse at CGRP. Now, more than 30 years later, migraine patients are prescribed CGRP antagonists.

In 1988, the first edition of the *International Classification of Headache Disorders* was published and, over 30 years later, the third edition has been published. This has enhanced migraine diagnostic criteria and refined our ability to conduct high-quality migraine research.

According to the Precision Medicine Initiative, precision medicine is "an emerging approach for disease treatment and prevention that takes into account individual variability in genes, environment and lifestyle for each person." This is totally consistent with how migraine patients should presently be evaluated and treated optimally.

This is in striking contrast to a one-size-fits-all approach, which puts less emphasis on individual differences. Shoshana emphasized, from a patient's perspective, the importance of this one-of-a-kind migraine patient and provider relationship. If accomplished routinely, it should result in a better understanding of unmet individual, diagnostic and treatment needs.

As we approach and hopefully embrace the future of migraine, we should always consider patient-dependent differences. The January 15, 2017, issue of *The New Yorker* published a patient-oriented article skillfully written by Atul Gawande, MD, MPH, a surgeon at Brigham and Women's Hospital in Boston, entitled "The Heroism of Incremental Care."

The article effectively and appropriately conveys that successful patient outcomes in nonsurgical areas of medicine, such as migraine, frequently require years to achieve. He denoted this time- and labor-intensive process as incremental care and contrasted its slow-but-steady improvement with surgery, which he defined as, "a definitive intervention at a critical moment in a person's life, with a clear, calculable, frequently transformative outcome." Dr. Gawande's article discusses a disabled chronic migraine patient whom Elizabeth Loder, MD, MPH evaluated. Dr. Loder is a neurologist and international thought leader in migraine and Chief, Division of Headache and Pain at the John R. Graham Headache Center in Boston. Dr. Gawande observed this evaluation and describes it as, "attentive and unhurried. She projected both professional confidence and maternal concern." He described this methodical attention to the patient's initial evaluation and subsequent visits, once again, as incremental care.

Establishing realistic migraine treatment goals and articulating them to patients has helped many of my patients achieve incremental success. There is no panacea or "silver bullet" for migraine; therefore, the systematic step-by-step process of incremental care applies to millions of migraine patients, and if applied appropriately, should result in a better future for millions of people who experience the pain and disability of migraine.

The continued evolution of our understanding of migraine diagnosis, epidemiology, pathophysiology and unmet treatment needs will continue to solidify the fact that migraine is a disabling, extremely prevalent, worldwide, neurologic disorder that should be diagnosed and treated optimally. All involved with migraine should be aware of the tremendous educational and patient-oriented support resources readily available and take advantage of these offerings.

I foresee a bright light, preferably when one no longer is light sensitive, at the end of the seemingly vast, all too often dark and dismal tunnel for all — by providing the right treatment to the right patient at the right time to optimally prevent and cure migraine. After all, migraine freedom is the Holy Grail and ultimate goal for all migraine patients.

Migraine in the Future
Patient's Perspective

Personally, I'm more hopeful about the future of migraine than I've ever been. Now, there is more awareness than ever — awareness that barely existed when I was first diagnosed in 1998.

With more awareness comes more understanding, sympathy, research, resources and treatment options. In 1998, I felt alone in my migraine struggles. Not anymore.

As we continue to learn more about migraine, patients are finally being recognized as the unique migraine sufferers we are. There's more willingness and openness from doctors to treat the individual and each patient's individual migraine. It's a relief.

I'm big on managing expectations — mine and others' — so understanding that there is no quick-fix migraine cure-all is important. As we've written about, there's a lot of trial and error, which I've experienced, but it has led to my incremental success.

Over the years, I have certainly had improvements in my migraine health — due to symptomatic and preventative medications and being aware of triggers and lifestyle changes — all of which have also evolved over the years. And I also have a better understanding of how I'm affected by migraine, which allows me to manage my situation better. When my body speaks, I listen. And thanks to Dr. Landy and available resources and tools, I'm better educated and equipped to handle it all.

Get educated. Communicate openly with your doctor. That should afford migraine sufferers the one-two punch needed to help them have healthier, less painful lives.

There's still more to do to help the one billion migraine sufferers around the globe. We're still in pain — though, hopefully, those days are significantly fewer than healthy days. New preventative and symptomatic treatment options would be welcome. The three new preventative injections are certainly terrific progress. And now, I see a nice, soft light slowly overtaking the darkness of migraine. It can only get even better from here.

Again, here's to your good health now and in the future.

"I fight for my health every day in ways most people don't understand. Hopefully, it'll continue to get a little easier going forward."

About the Author

STEPHEN LANDY, MD, FAAN, FAHS, is a neurologist who's practiced headache medicine for over 30 years. He directs Landy Headache & Esthetics in Tupelo, Mississippi, and is a Clinical Professor of Neurology at the University of Tennessee Medical School. 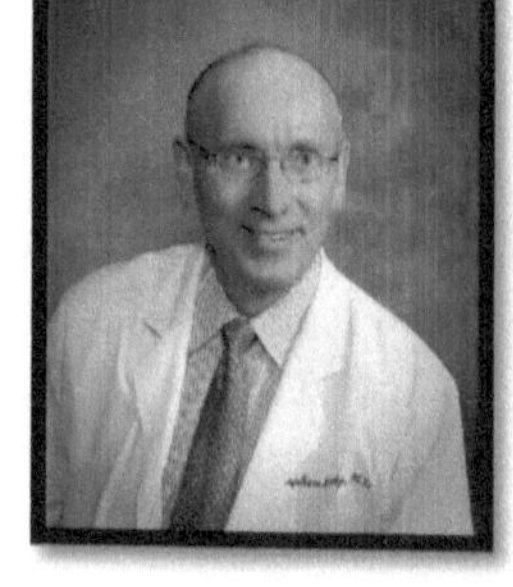

Dr. Landy graduated from the University of Tennessee Medical School and completed his neurology residency at Vanderbilt University. He is board certified in neurology and headache medicine and is a Fellow of the American Academy of Neurology and American Headache Society.

Dr. Landy has two sons, both physicians, and resides in Tupelo, MS with his wife Leighann and her two children. His pastimes include sports, music, reading, and spending time with his family.

About the Author

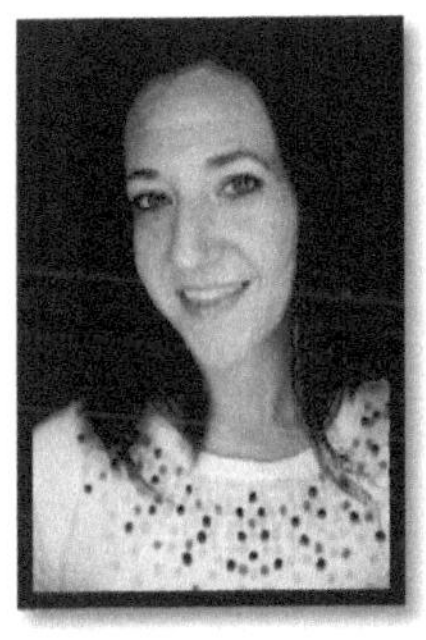

SHOSHANA Y. CENKER is a professional content writer, editor, proofreader, copywriter, marketing consultant, wordsmith extraordinaire and word & grammar nerd. A communications specialist, if you will.

She and her three young kiddos — 9-year-old twin boys Aiden and Akiva, and 7-year-old daughter Lyla — live in her hometown of Memphis, TN. Shoshana enjoys traveling, cooking, karaoke, musicals and working out. She especially loves spending time being active with her kids at parks, on hikes, roller skating, biking around their neighborhood and walking their pups, Dreidel and Memphis.

HEAD CASE

Thank you so much for shedding some light on the darkness of migraines with your story "Peace of Mind" [by Daryl Chen, photographed by Irving Penn, May]. At 24, I've been suffering from them for six years. My friends didn't really understand how debilitating the condition is until I was rushed to the hospital one afternoon. The more informed people are, the better they can understand what we go through.

Shoshana Yaffe
Silver Spring, MD

Shoshana's Letter to the Editor published in *Vogue Magazine* August 2004

APPENDIX

Pertinent Publications

The Migraine Enigma

1. S. Landy. The Man With Headache and Weakness (Hemiplegic Migraine). In: Tepper SJ, Sheftell F, Rapoport AM, eds. The Spectrum of Migraine. Pages 116-122. McMahon Publishing Group. New York, NY. 2002.

2. S. Landy. Acute Treatment Goals in Migraine: Expanding the Diagnosis and Treatment of Migraine. 2003;*Medscape*: www.medscape.com.

3. S. Landy. Migraine Headaches and Allodynia: Early Use of Triptans to Improve Outcome. 2003;*Medscape*: www.medscape.com.

4. S. Landy, et al. Headache in the Workplace: An Evaluation of the Impact of Educational Programming on Employee Disability. *Headache & Pain*. 2003;14:156-160.

5. S. Landy. Migraine Throughout the Life cycle. Treatment through the Ages. *Neurology*. 2004;62 (Suppl 2):82-88.

6. S. Landy. Central Sensitisation and Cutaneous Allodynia in Migraine: Implications for Treatment. *CNS Drugs*. 2004;18:337-342.

7. S. Landy, et al. Migraine: A Better Way to Recognize and Treat It. A Prospective Study Shows How the

Migraine Care Program Makes Management Easier and Improves Patient Satisfaction. *The Journal of Family Practice.* 2006;55,1038-1047.

8. S. Landy, et al. Clarification of Developing and Established Clinical Allodynia and Pain-Free Outcomes. *Headache.* 2007;47:247-252.

9. S. Landy, et al. A Migraine Disease Management Program in the Primary Care Setting: Impact on Patient Quality of Life and Productivity Loss. *Journal of Clinical Outcomes Management.* 2007;14:332-338.

10. S. Landy, et al. Examining the Interrelationship of Migraine Onset, Duration, and Time to Treatment. *Headache.* 2012;52:363-373.

My Migraine Journey
The Migraine Enigma